Diabetes Juicing Cookbook

Delicious and Nutritious Diabetes Juicing Diet

Melanie Dobbins

Copyright © [2023], [Melanie Dobbins]

Table of Contents

INTRODUCTION

Sylvia has been attempting nearly every therapy option for her diabetes without much success for many years. She was depressed and feeling dismal about her situation, and she was on the verge of giving up.

She came across one of my social media articles describing a unique juicing diet that might be able to reverse diabetes one day. She was initially dubious, but in need of a fix, she decided to give it a shot.

The diet was straightforward but rigid. She was required to drink six tiny juices made from fruits and vegetables each day. The juices had all organic components and were low in sugar while being high in nutrients.

Sylvia first had her doubts about the diet and feared that it wouldn't be successful. Yet after a few weeks, she noticed a change in her level of energy and general wellness.

Within a few months, Sylvia was feeling better than she had in years. Her blood sugar levels returned to normal, and her diabetes had completely resolved. She was so pleased with the outcomes that she decided to continue the diet and reap the rewards.

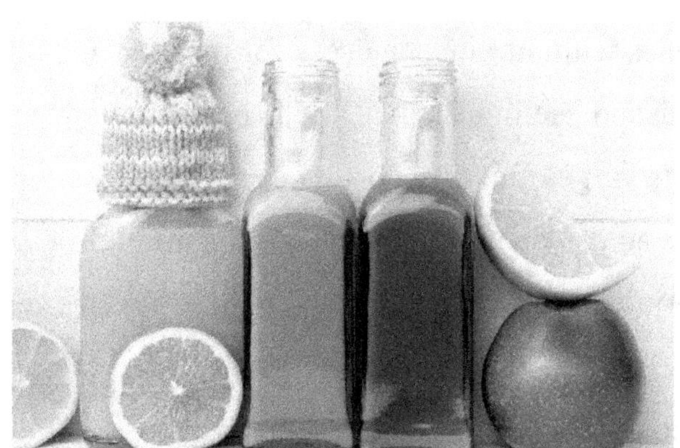

Sylvia was astounded by how much her life had altered as a result of beginning the juicing diet. She was energized and loving life once more. She was happy to have discovered a remedy that worked for her and vowed to spread the word about the effectiveness of juicing in reversing diabetes.

Sylvia's story of achievement served as a sign of hope for other diabetics. She served as living proof that the appropriate juicing diet might significantly improve the lives of people suffering from this crippling condition.

Juicing for diabetes

Consuming freshly produced juice from fruits and vegetables as part of a diabetes care regimen is known as diabetes juicing. Diabetics can obtain the essential vitamins and nutrients they need to help control their diabetes by sipping fresh juice.

Rules for Juicing for Diabetes

1. To obtain the most nutrition and benefit from your juices, make sure to include a range of low-sugar fruits and vegetables. Diabetics should strive to consume a variety of fruits and vegetables in their juices. For diabetics, low-sugar foods including spinach, celery, cucumber, kale, and grapefruit are especially advantageous.

2. Refrain from adding extra sugar: Juices for diabetics shouldn't contain any extra sugar or sweeteners. Even organic sweets like honey and maple syrup should be avoided because they can increase blood sugar levels.

3. Immediately after making the juice, consume it. This will ensure that you obtain the most amount of nourishment from

the juice. Store it in the fridge for up to 24 hours if it can't be eaten right away.

4. Take into account include supplements: Using supplements like omega-3 fatty acids, probiotics, and vitamins can boost the juice's nutritional worth. Which supplements are most suitable for a specific person can be decided with the aid of a healthcare practitioner.

Benefits of Juicing for Diabetes

1. **Better blood sugar control:** Juice's low glycemic index can help balance blood sugar levels when consumed. For diabetics who must maintain control over their blood sugar levels, this can be extremely helpful.

2. **Improved nutritional intake:** Fruits and vegetables can be juiced to give concentrated forms of antioxidants, vitamins, and minerals that can support optimum health.

3. **Better kidney health:** Juicing can help diabetics' kidneys function more efficiently and lower their chances of developing kidney disease.

4. **Lower risk of complications:** Drinking freshly prepared juice can help lower the risk of complications from diabetes, including heart disease, stroke, and blindness. You can also check my book for more healthy ways to maintain your blood sugar levels here

5. **Weight management:** Because some juices are low in calories and can assist to reduce cravings for unhealthy foods, juicing can also support weight management in diabetics.

Overall, managing diabetes and enhancing general health can be accomplished with diabetic juicing. To maximize the

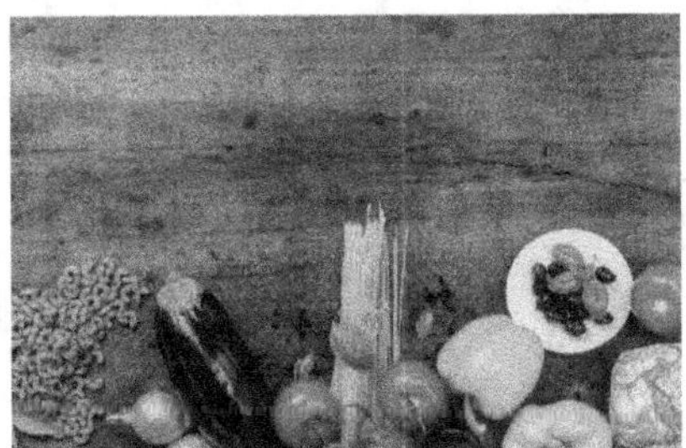

benefits, it's crucial to abide by the guidelines listed above and never consume more juice than is advised in a day.

BEST FRUITS AND VEGETABLES FOR DIABETES JUICING

1. **Carrots**: Rich in potassium, manganese, fiber, and vitamins A, B6, C, and K, carrots are a fantastic source of vitamins and minerals. Carrots are a fantastic food option for diabetics since their fiber content helps slow down the absorption of sugar into the system. In addition to being fat-free and low in calories, carrots are a fantastic supplement to any diabetes juicing routine.

2. **Celery**: Celery is a low-calorie vegetable that is rich in fiber, potassium, manganese, vitamins A, B6, C, and K, as well as other nutrients. Dietary fiber, which is abundant in celery, aids in digestion control and helps to slow down the absorption of sugar into the bloodstream. Celery is a fantastic source of antioxidants, which can help guard against issues associated with diabetes.

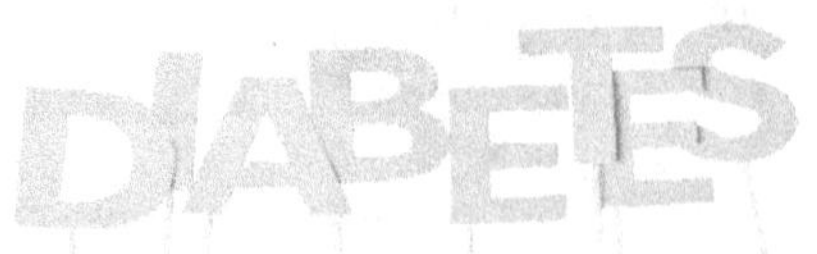

3. **Beets**: Beets are a great source of fiber, potassium, manganese, and vitamins A, B6, C, and K. Moreover, beets are a strong source of folate, which lowers the risk of some birth abnormalities. The fiber component of beets helps to slow down the absorption of sugar into the bloodstream and can assist to manage blood sugar levels.

4. **Spinach**: A, B6, C, and K vitamins, as well as potassium, manganese, and fiber are all abundant in spinach. Lutein and zeaxanthin, two significant antioxidants that can help to stave off eye issues associated with diabetes, are also abundant in spinach. Spinach is a great complement to any diabetes juicing routine because it has few calories and no fat.

5. **Cucumbers**: In addition to potassium, manganese, and fiber, cucumbers are a fantastic source of vitamins A, B6, C, and K. In addition to being low in calories and fat, cucumbers are a fantastic option for diabetics. Cucumbers include fiber, which helps to control digestion and slow down the absorption of sugar into the bloodstream.

Cucumbers are high in water, which might help you stay hydrated and lose weight.

6. **Tomatoes**: Tomatoes are a great source of potassium, manganese, fiber, and vitamins A, B6, C, and K. Lycopene, a potent antioxidant that can help to prevent diabetes-related problems, is another important component of tomatoes. Given their low calorie and fat content, tomatoes are a fantastic addition to any diabetes juicing routine.

7. **Apples**: Apples are a rich source of potassium, manganese, fiber, and vitamins A, B6, C, and K. Pectin is a soluble fiber that serves to slow down the absorption of sugar into the bloodstream and is abundant in apples. Apples are a fantastic option for diabetics because they have few calories and no fat.

8. **Blueberries**: Excellent sources of potassium, manganese, fiber, and vitamins A, B6, C, and K may be found in blueberries. Antioxidant-rich blueberries can aid in preventing diabetes-related problems. In addition to being

fat-free and low in calories, blueberries are a fantastic complement to any diabetes juicing routine.

9. **Strawberries**: Excellent sources of potassium, manganese, fiber, and vitamins A, B6, C, and K may be found in strawberries. Antioxidants found in strawberries are also a wonderful source of defense against difficulties brought on by diabetes. Strawberries are a fantastic food option for diabetics because they are low in calories and fat-free.

10. **Kale**: Kale is a great source of potassium, manganese, fiber, and vitamins A, B6, C, and K. In addition, kale contains significant amounts of lutein and zeaxanthin, two potent antioxidants that can help guard against eye issues brought on by diabetes.

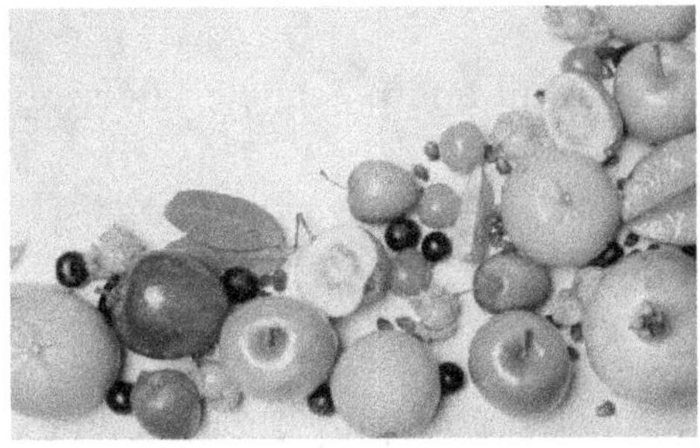

DIABETES JUICING RECIPES

Grapefruit and Pineapple Juice

Ingredients

- 1/2 large grapefruit, peeled and roughly chopped
- 1/2 cup fresh or frozen pineapple chunks
- 1 tablespoon freshly grated ginger
- 1 tablespoon honey (optional)
- 1 cup cold water

Instructions:

1. Combine the grapefruit, pineapple, ginger, honey (if using), and water in a blender.
2. Blend until smooth.
3. Pour the mixture through a fine-mesh strainer into a bowl or cup.
4. Serve the grapefruit and pineapple juice immediately or chill until ready to serve.

Tips:

- Make sure to peel and roughly chop the grapefruit before blending for a smoother texture.

- For sweeter juice, add a bit more honey.

- If the juice is too tart, add a splash of freshly-squeezed orange juice.

- To make a slushy, freeze the juice in an ice cube tray and blend until smooth.

- For spicier juice, add a pinch of cayenne pepper or a small piece of jalapeno.

- If you don't have fresh pineapple, you can use canned or frozen pineapple.

- If you don't have fresh ginger, you can use ground ginger.

- To make it a cocktail, add a splash of vodka or white rum.

- If you need to make a larger batch, simply double or triple the recipe.

- For lighter juice, replace the water with sparkling water or seltzer.

- For creamier juice, add a few tablespoons of coconut cream.

- To make a slushy, blend the juice with a handful of ice cubes.

- For frothy juice, blend the juice with an immersion blender or use a milk frothier.

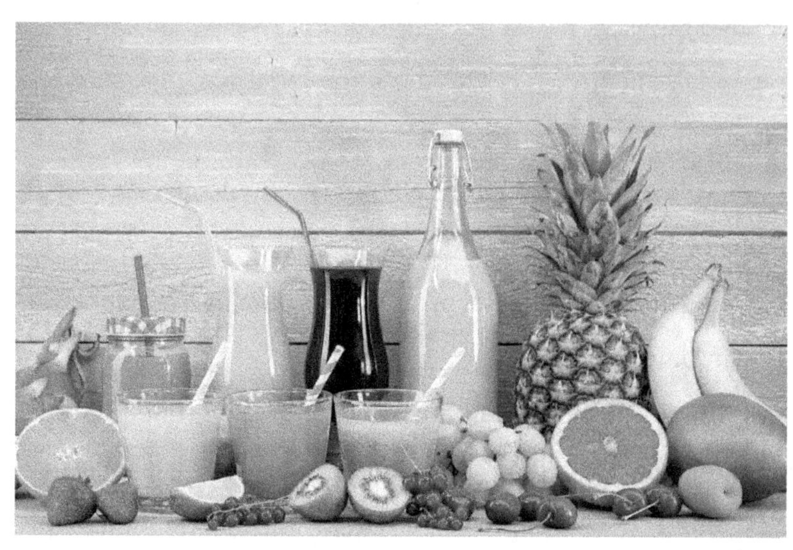

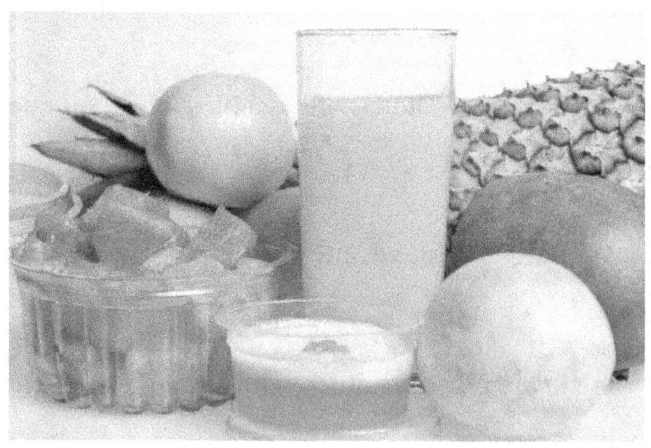

Cucumber and Kale Juice

Ingredients:

- 2 cucumbers

- 2 cups kale

- 1 lemon

- 1-inch piece of ginger

- 1 tablespoon honey (optional)

Instructions:

1. Wash the cucumbers and kale thoroughly.

2. Peel the cucumbers and cut them into cubes.

3. Remove the stems from the kale and break them into small pieces.

4. Peel the ginger and cut it into thin slices.

5. Squeeze the juice from the lemon.

6. Place the cucumber cubes, kale, ginger, lemon juice, and honey (if using) into a blender and blend until smooth.

7. Strain the juice through a fine mesh sieve and discard the pulp.

8. Pour the juice into glasses and enjoy!

Tips:

- You can add a few ice cubes to the juice to make it colder.

- If you don't like the taste of honey, you can add a few drops of stevia or agave syrup instead.

- You can also add other greens such as spinach, celery, or parsley to the juice for a nutritional boost.

- For a refreshing twist, add a few mints leaves to the juice.

- If you would like to make the juice thicker, you can add a banana or avocado to the blender.

- If you want to make the juice sweeter, you can add some apple or pineapple juice.

- You can store the juice in the refrigerator for up to 3 days.

- If you have a juicer, you can use it instead of a blender to make the juice.

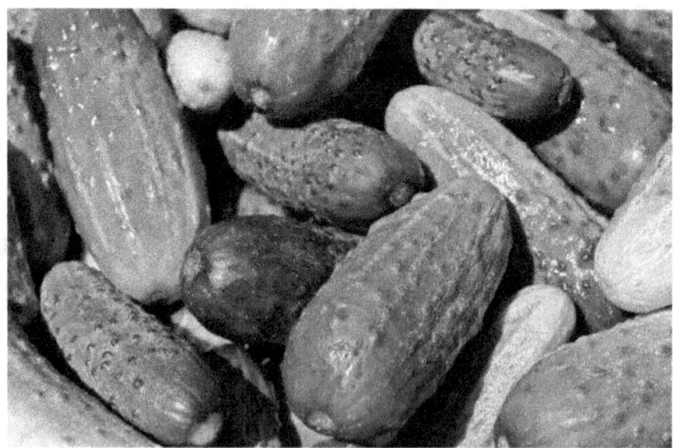

Protein Boost Juice

Ingredients:

- 1 cup of kale, chopped

- 1 cup of spinach, chopped

- 1 banana, peeled and sliced

- 1 cup of almond milk

- ½ cup of plain yogurt

- 2 tablespoons of ground flaxseed

Instructions:

1. Put the kale and spinach into a blender and blend until smooth.

2. Add the banana, almond milk, yogurt, and flaxseed and blend until mixed.

3. Pour the juice into a glass and enjoy!

Tips:

- For sweeter juice, add honey or maple syrup to taste.

- Add a scoop of protein powder to increase the protein content.

- You can also add some ice cubes to make it more refreshing.

- For a thicker consistency, add more yogurt or almond milk.

- To make it more nutritious, add other superfoods such as chia seeds and hemp seeds.

- If you don't have fresh kale and spinach, you can use frozen instead.

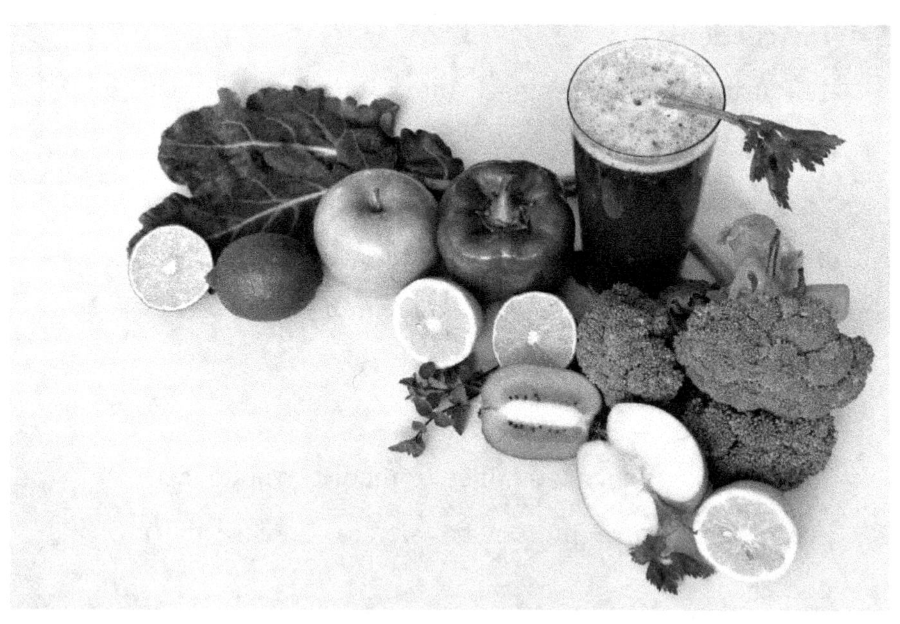

Beetroot and Orange Juice

Ingredients:

- 2 large beets, peeled and cut into cubes

- 2 oranges, peeled and cubed

- 2 carrots, peeled and sliced

- 2 celery stalks, chopped

- 1-inch piece of ginger, peeled and grated

- 2 cups of water

- 2 tablespoons of honey (optional)

Instructions:

1. Place the beets, oranges, carrots, celery, and ginger in a blender or food processor.

2. Add the water and blend until the ingredients are fully combined and the mixture is smooth.

3. If desired, add honey to the juice for a sweeter taste.

4. Strain the juice through a fine mesh strainer to remove any pulp or chunks.

5. Serve the Beetroot and Orange Juice immediately or store in the refrigerator for up to 2 days.

Tips:

- For a frothier, creamier juice, add a handful of ice cubes to the blender.

- For spicier juice, add a pinch of cayenne pepper or a dash of hot sauce.

- If you're looking for an additional nutrient boost, add a handful of spinach or kale to the blender.

- If you want to make the juice sweeter, add a few drops of stevia or a teaspoon of maple syrup.

- If you want to make the juice less sweet, try adding a squeeze of lemon juice or a splash of apple cider vinegar.

- Make sure to use organic produce to get the best-tasting and healthiest juice.

- If you're using pre-cut beets and oranges, make sure to rinse them thoroughly before using them.

- If you want to make a larger batch of juice, simply double or triple the ingredients.

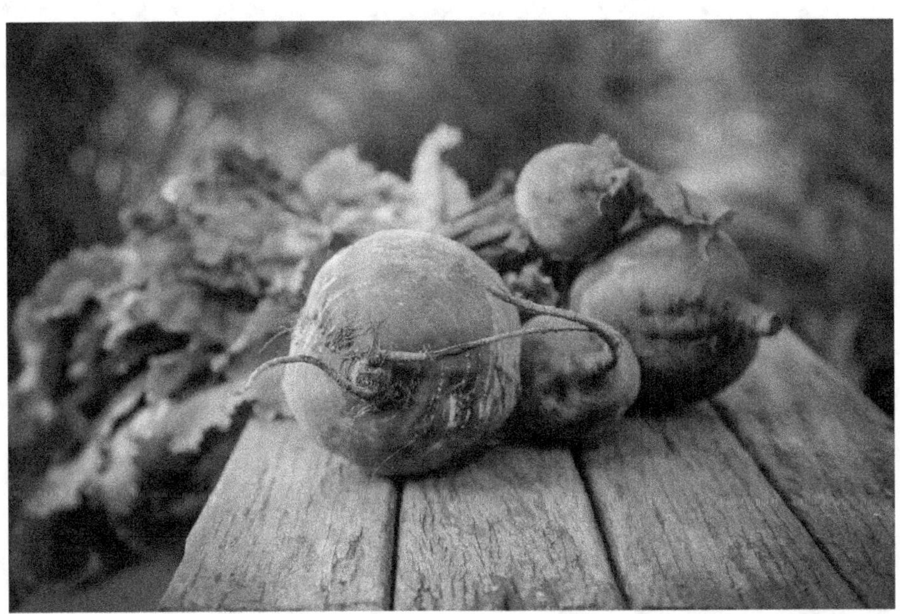

Green Juice

Ingredients:

- 4-5 stalks of celery
- 1 cucumber
- 1 handful of kale
- 1 handful of spinach
- 2 apples
- 1 inch of fresh ginger

Instructions:

1. Wash all the produce thoroughly before beginning.
2. Peel the ginger and cut it into smaller pieces.
3. Chop the celery, cucumber, and apples into smaller pieces.
4. Add all the produce to a blender or juicer.
5. Blend or juice for 1-2 minutes until all the ingredients are combined.
6. Enjoy your green juice!

Tips:

- You can adjust the ingredients to your liking. For example, if you don't like the taste of kale, you can reduce the amount or leave it out entirely.

- If you are using a blender, you can add a cup of water or coconut water to make it smoother.

- You can also add a tablespoon of honey or another sweetener to make the juice more palatable.

- If you are using a juicer, you can save the pulp and use it in smoothies or as a topping on salads.

- Drink the juice right away for maximum health benefits.

- If you are not going to drink the juice immediately, store it in an airtight container and drink it within 24 hours.

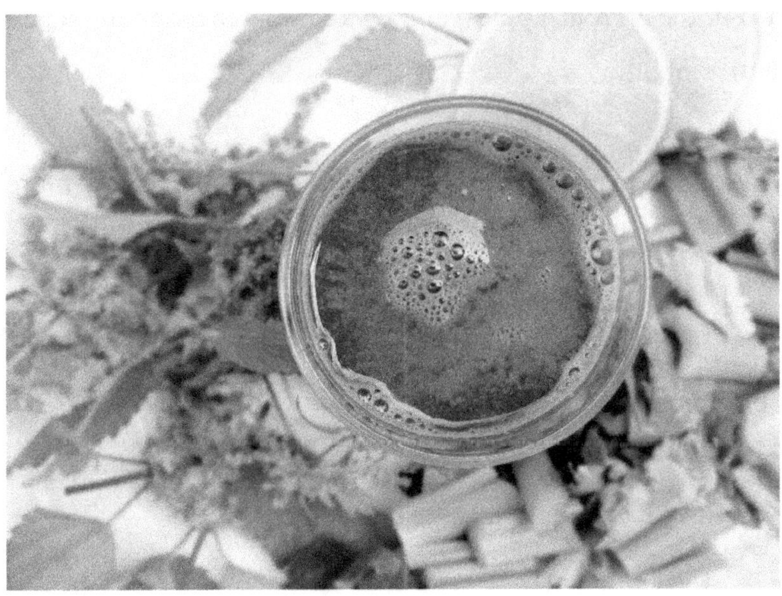

Carrot and Apple Juice

Ingredients

- 3 large carrots, peeled and chopped

- 2 large apples, cored and chopped

- 2 tablespoons of freshly squeezed lemon juice

- 1 teaspoon of freshly grated ginger

- 2 cups of water

Instructions

1. Put the carrots, apples, and water into a blender and blend until smooth.

2. Add the lemon juice and ginger and blend for a few more seconds until everything is well incorporated.

3. Strain the juice through a fine mesh sieve to remove any solid pieces.

4. Pour the juice into glasses and serve.

Tips

- For sweeter juice, add a tablespoon of honey.

- You can also add a pinch of ground cinnamon or nutmeg for a more complex flavor.

- If you prefer a thicker juice, you can add some ice cubes to the blender or strain the juice through a cheesecloth or nut milk bag.

- For a more nutritious juice, add a handful of baby spinach or kale.

- You can also add other fruits such as oranges, pineapple, or mangoes to your juice.

- If you want to add more flavor, you can add a teaspoon of freshly squeezed ginger juice.

- To make a smoothie, you can add a few tablespoons of your favorite yogurt or some frozen bananas.

- If you are using store-bought juice, make sure it is 100% juice and not from concentrate.

- You can also add some fresh herbs such as basil or mint to your juice.

- If you prefer a less pulpy juice, you can strain it through a cheesecloth or nut milk bag.

- If you are using apples, make sure you are using sweet apples such as Honey crisp or Gala.

- If you want to make a larger batch of juice, you can double

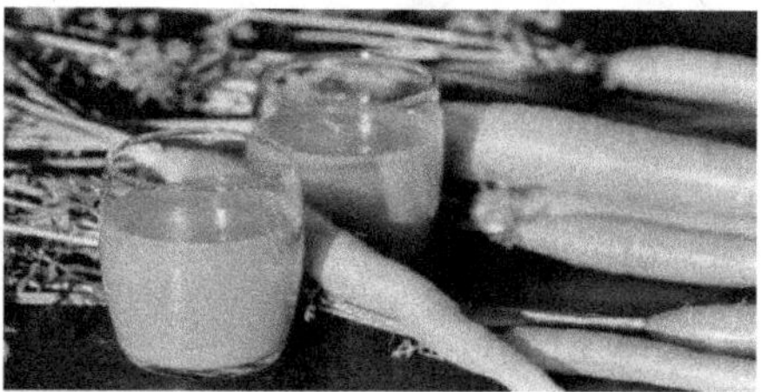

or triple the ingredients.

- Keep in mind that the juice will separate over time, so be sure to give it a good shake before serving.

- Store leftovers in an airtight container in the refrigerator for up to 3 days.

Blueberry and Pear Juice

Ingredients:

- 2 cups fresh blueberries
- 2 pears, cored and chopped
- 1/2 cup freshly squeezed lemon juice
- 2 tablespoons honey
- 2 cups cold water

Instructions:

1. Place the blueberries, pears, and lemon juice in a blender and blend on high speed until smooth.

2. Add the honey and water to the blender and blend again until combined.

3. Strain the mixture through a fine mesh sieve or cheesecloth to remove any solids.

4. Pour the juice into glasses and serve.

Tips:

- For a sweeter juice, add more honey to taste.

- If you like a thicker juice, add 1/4 cup of chia seeds for added thickness.

- You can also add a pinch of cinnamon or ginger for an extra flavor kick.

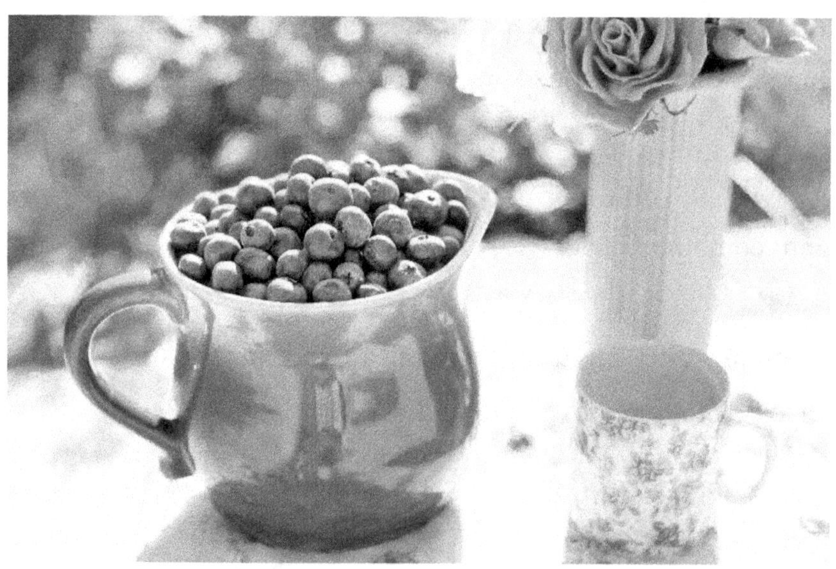

Bloody Mary Juice

Ingredients:

- 2 large beets, peeled and cut into large cubes

- 2 carrots, peeled and cut into large cubes

- 2 stalks of celery, chopped

- 4 large tomatoes, quartered

- 2 tablespoons Worcestershire sauce

- 1 teaspoon horseradish

- 2 tablespoons freshly squeezed lemon juice

- 1 teaspoon freshly ground black pepper

- 1 teaspoon celery salt

Instructions:

1. In a large pot, combine the beets, carrots, celery, tomatoes, Worcestershire sauce, horseradish, and 1 cup of water.

2. Bring to a boil, reduce the heat to low, and simmer for 15 minutes.

3. Use an immersion blender or a food processor, blend the mixture until smooth.

4. Strain the mixture through a fine mesh strainer into a large bowl.

5. Add the lemon juice, black pepper, and celery salt, and stir to combine.

6. Serve immediately.

Tips:

- For an extra kick, add a splash of hot sauce or vodka to your Bloody Mary juice.

- For a spicier version, try adding some freshly grated ginger

- If you prefer a sweeter taste, add a tablespoon of honey or agave syrup.

- For a thicker consistency, use less water or add a small amount of tomato paste.

- To make a thicker version of the juice, use a potato masher to mash the vegetables before blending.

- For a more savory flavor, try adding a few cloves of garlic.

- If you like your Bloody Mary juice a bit tangier, add a few tablespoons of apple cider vinegar.

- For a smoky flavor, try adding a few tablespoons of smoked paprika.

- If you like a stronger horseradish flavor, add an extra teaspoon of horseradish.

- Garnish your Bloody Mary juice with celery, cucumber, olives, or pickles.

- For an extra layer of flavor, try adding a few dashes of Worcestershire sauce.

- If you want a more exotic flavor, add a teaspoon of cardamom or coriander.

Watermelon and Mint Juice

Ingredients:

- 2 cups of cubed watermelon

- 1/4 cup of fresh mint leaves

- 1/4 cup of freshly squeezed lime juice

- 1/4 cup of cold water

- 1 to 2 tablespoons of honey or agave syrup (optional)

Instructions:

1. Place the cubed watermelon in a blender and blend until smooth.

2. Add the mint leaves and blend for another 30 seconds.

3. Add the lime juice, water, and honey or agave syrup (optional) and blend until all ingredients are fully incorporated.

4. Strain the mixture through a fine-mesh strainer into a pitcher.

5. Serve over ice and enjoy!

Tips:

- Make sure to use ripe, juicy watermelon for the best results.

- If you don't have a strainer, you can use a cheesecloth to strain out any large chunks of watermelon.

- Feel free to adjust the amount of honey or agave syrup according to your taste preferences.

- For a more refreshing flavor, add a few slices of fresh lime and a few extra mint leaves to the pitcher before serving.

- If you're feeling adventurous, try adding a pinch of chili powder or a few drops of Tabasco sauce for a unique twist on the classic recipe.

- For a thicker consistency, add a few cubes of frozen watermelon when blending.

- For a more tropical flavor, try substituting some of the water with pineapple juice or coconut water.

- To make a more health-conscious version of the drink, replace the honey or agave syrup with stevia or monk fruit.

- If you're making a larger batch of the juice, you can refrigerate the mixture for up to three days.

- If you plan on serving the juice in individual glasses, feel free to garnish each glass with a few extra mint leaves or a slice of fresh lime.

- For a boozy twist, replace the water with your favorite white rum or vodka.

- If you're looking to make a mocktail version of the drink, replace the water with sparkling water or ginger beer.

- Feel free to experiment with different types of watermelons, such as yellow or orange, for a unique flavor.

- You can use frozen watermelon for the recipe, but make sure to thaw it out before blending.

- If you're not a fan of mint, you can substitute it with fresh basil or cilantro.

- If you're looking for a vegan version of the drink, simply replace the honey or agave syrup with your favorite plant-based sweetener.

- For a more decadent version of the juice, try adding a scoop of your favorite ice cream or yogurt for a creamy texture.

- You can also freeze the juice in an ice cube tray to make delicious and refreshing ice cubes for smoothies or other drinks.

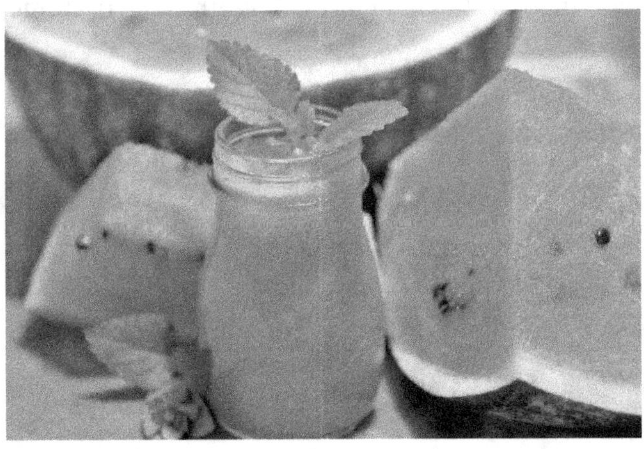

Carrot and Celery Juice

Ingredients:

-2 cups of chopped carrots

-2 cups of chopped celery

-½ lemon, juiced

-2 cups of water (optional)

Instructions:

1. Wash, peel, and chop the carrots and celery into small pieces.

2. Place the chopped carrots and celery in a blender or food processor.

3. Add the lemon juice and water (if desired).

4. Blend the ingredients until a smooth juice is formed.

5. Pour the juice into a glass and enjoy!

Tips:

• If you want to add a bit of sweetness, you can add a bit of honey or agave nectar to the juice.

• For a bit of a kick, you can add a few slices of ginger or a pinch of cayenne pepper to the juice.

• For thicker juice, you can add a few ice cubes to the blender before blending.

• You can also add other fruits and vegetables to the juice, such as apples, oranges, spinach, kale, etc.

• You can also add some Greek yogurt to make the juice creamier.

• If you want to make the juice more nutritious, you can add some chia seeds or flax seeds.

• If you don't have a blender or food processor, you can use a hand-held juicer to make the juice.

• The juice can be stored in the refrigerator for up to 3 days.

• You can also freeze the juice in an airtight container for up to 3 months.

• For an extra boost of nutrition, you can add some protein powder or superfoods to the juice.

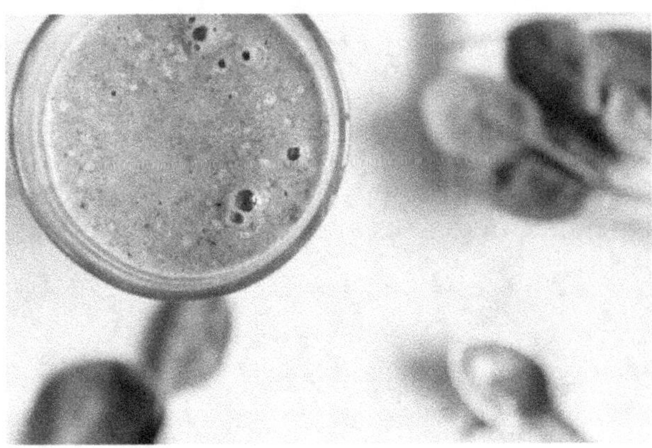

Mango and Papaya Juice

Ingredients:

-2 ripe mangoes

-1 ripe papaya

-2 limes

-2 cups of ice

Instructions:

1. Peel and cut both mangoes and papaya into small pieces.

2. Place the mango and papaya pieces in a blender, and add the juice of two limes.

3. Blend the mixture until it is smooth.

4. Add the ice to the blender and blend again until the ice is crushed.

5. Serve the juice in glasses and enjoy!

Tips:

• If you don't have access to ripe mangoes and papaya, you can substitute with frozen mango and papaya pieces.

• For a sweeter taste, add a tablespoon of honey or sugar to the mix before blending.

• To make a refreshing smoothie instead of juice, add a cup of yogurt or milk to the blend.

• For a more exotic flavor, add a pinch of ground ginger or cardamom to the mix before blending.

• If you have leftover juice, store it in the refrigerator and enjoy it within a few days.

• To make the juice even healthier, add a handful of spinach or kale to the mix before blending.

• If you're not a fan of lime juice, you can substitute it with orange or pineapple juice.

• To make the juice more nutritious, blend in a few tablespoons of chia or flax seeds.

• Enjoy the juice with a sprinkle of fresh mint leaves for an even more refreshing taste.

• For a more tropical flavor, add a few slices of fresh pineapple to the blend.

• If you'd like to make the juice even creamier, blend in a few tablespoons of almond or coconut milk.

• For a boozy version of the juice, add a shot of dark rum or tequila to the mix before blending.

• For a vegan alternative, substitute the yogurt or milk with coconut yogurt or almond milk.

• For an extra kick, add a pinch of cayenne pepper to the mix before blending.

• To make the juice more filling, add a few tablespoons of oats or quinoa to the blend.

• To make the juice more nutrient-dense, blend in a scoop of your favorite protein powder.

• Enjoy the juice with a few slices of fresh fruit for an even more delicious flavor.

• Don't forget to garnish the glasses with a few slices of fresh mango or papaya for a beautiful presentation.

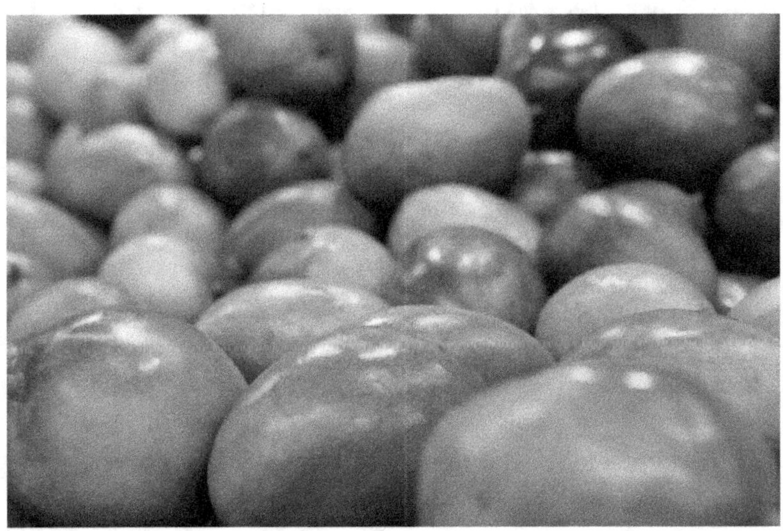

Mexican Juice

Ingredients:

-2 ripe avocados

-1 jalapeno, seeded and minced

-1/4 cup cilantro, finely chopped

-2 limes, juiced

-2 tomatoes, diced

-1/4 red onion, diced

Instructions:

1. Start by preparing the vegetables. Peel the avocados and remove the pits. Cut them into small cubes. Mince the jalapeno, chop the cilantro, dice the tomatoes, and dice the red onion.

2. Place all of the vegetables into a blender.

3. Squeeze the juice of 2 limes into the blender.

4. Blend until all of the ingredients are well combined.

5. Taste and adjust the flavor to your preference.

6. Serve in a glass with ice cubes and a wedge of lime.

Tips:

-For a spicier juice, add more jalapeno or leave some of the seeds in.

-If you want a more savory juice, add a pinch of salt.

-You can also add some fresh mint leaves for a refreshing flavor.

-If you want a thicker juice, add a bit of avocado or Greek yogurt.

-If you want to add some sweetness, add a bit of honey or agave syrup.

-You can also add other vegetables such as bell peppers, cucumbers, or celery.

-For a creamier juice, blend in some coconut milk.

-You can also add a splash of orange juice for a fruity flavor.

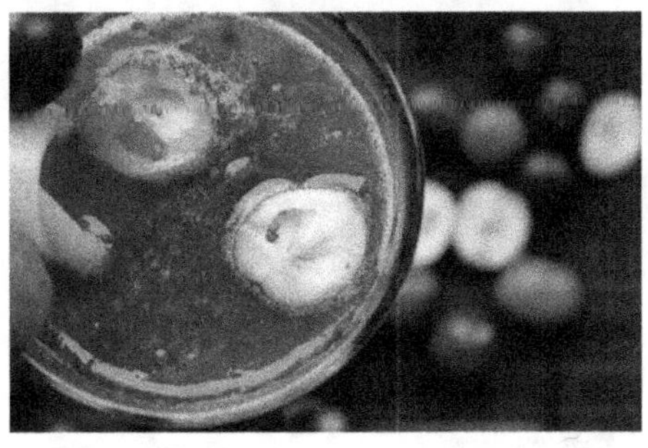

Apple and Beetroot Juice

Ingredients:

- 2 apples

- 1 beetroot

- 1/2 inch piece of ginger

- 1/2 lemon

- 1 cup of ice

- 2 tablespoons of honey (optional)

Instructions:

1. Peel and chop the apples into small pieces.

2. Peel and grate the beetroot.

3. Peel and grate the ginger.

4. Squeeze the lemon juice.

5. Combine the apples, beetroot, ginger, and lemon juice in a blender.

6. Blend until smooth.

7. Add the ice and honey (if desired) and blend again until smooth.

8. Pour the juice into a glass and enjoy!

Tips:

- For best results, use a high-powered blender.

- For a sweeter juice, add more honey or a few drops of stevia.

- If the juice is too thick, add a few tablespoons of water or coconut water.

- Adding a few sprigs of fresh mint will give the juice a nice flavor.

- If you don't have a lemon, substitute with a few drops of apple cider vinegar.

- Use organic ingredients whenever possible.

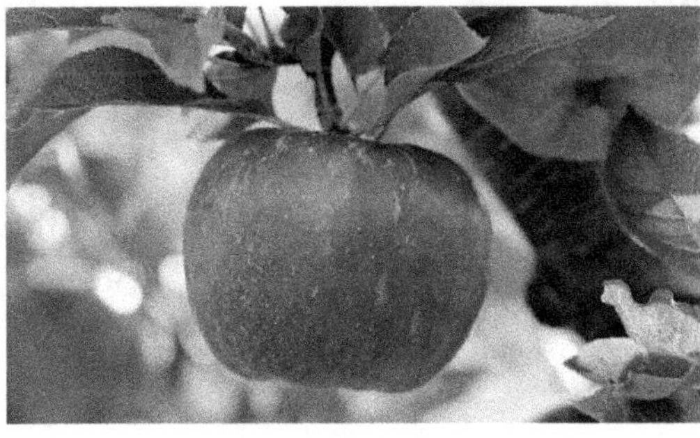

Orange and Carrot Juice

Ingredients:

- 2 oranges

- 2 carrots

- 2 tablespoons of lemon juice

- Ice (optional)

Instructions:

1. Peel the oranges and carrots.

2. Cut the carrots into small cubes and the oranges into slices.

3. Place the orange and carrot cubes into a blender.

4. Add the lemon juice to the blender.

5. Blend the mixture for about two minutes or until the ingredients are completely blended.

6. Pour the juice into a glass and add ice (optional).

7. Serve and enjoy!

Tips:

- For a more intense orange flavor, add a few drops of orange extract.

- You can also add a dash of sugar or honey to sweeten the juice.

- For an extra-refreshing drink, add a few mints leaves to the blender.

- You can also add some apples or other fruits to vary the flavor.

- If you want a smoother consistency, strain the juice before serving.

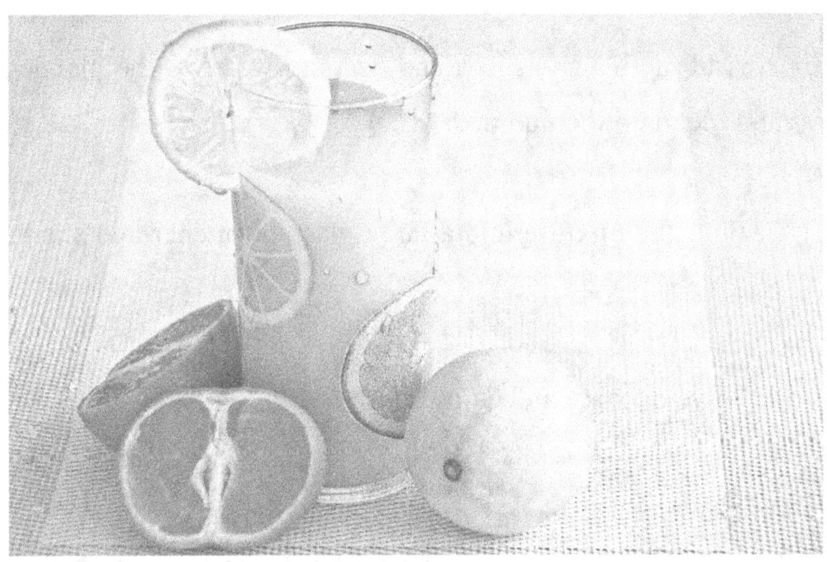

Pineapple and Banana Juice

Ingredients:

- 1 large fresh pineapple, peeled, cored, and cut into chunks
- 1 ripe banana, peeled and sliced
- 1 cup of coconut water

Instructions:

1. Place the pineapple chunks in a blender and blend until smooth.

2. Add the banana slices and coconut water to the blender and blend until combined.

3. Pour the mixture into a large glass or pitcher and stir to combine.

4. Serve over ice and enjoy!

Tips:

- To make sure your pineapple is ripe, look for one with a yellow-brown color and slightly soft to the touch.

- For an extra sweet treat, you can add a tablespoon of honey or maple syrup to the blender before blending.

- You can also add a splash of orange or lime juice for an extra zesty flavor.

- If you don't have fresh pineapple, you can use canned pineapple chunks, just make sure to drain them before adding them to the blender.

- If you want a thicker consistency, add a few ice cubes to the blender before blending.

- To make this a healthy smoothie, add a scoop of your favorite protein powder or a handful of spinach.

- You can also make this a frozen treat by blending the mixture with a few ice cubes before serving.

- To make a vegan or dairy-free version, use almond or coconut milk in place of the coconut water.

- If you want to make it even more tropical, add a scoop of mango or passion fruit puree before blending.

- This juice is also great with a little bit of freshly grated ginger or turmeric added before blending.

- You can also top your Pineapple and Banana Juice with a dollop of Greek yogurt or coconut cream for an extra creamy finish.

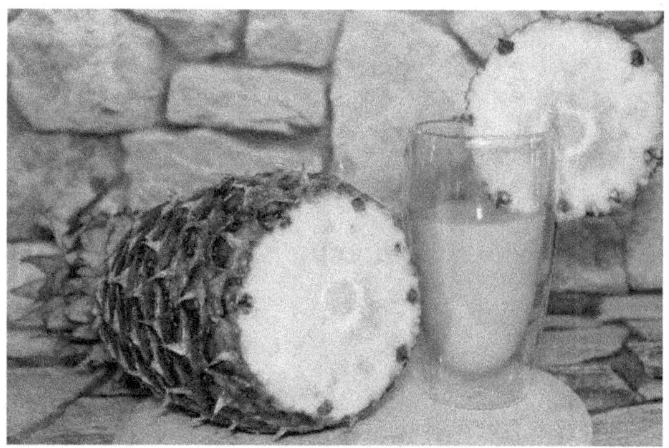

- If you want to make it extra special, add a sprinkle of freshly chopped mint or basil leaves before serving.

- For a decadent treat, top the juice with a few slices of freshly cut pineapple and a sprinkle of toasted coconut.

Strawberry and Spinach Juice

Ingredients:

-1 cup of fresh, sliced strawberries

-2 cups of fresh spinach

-1/4 cup of freshly squeezed lime juice

Instructions:

1. Wash the strawberries and spinach thoroughly to ensure they are free of dirt and debris.

2. Cut the stems off the strawberries and cut them into small pieces.

3. Place the strawberries and spinach into a blender or food processor.

4. Add the freshly squeezed lime juice and blend until the mixture is smooth.

5. Pour the juice into a glass and enjoy!

Tips:

-If you are not a fan of the tartness of the lime juice, you can substitute it with honey or agave syrup for a sweeter juice.

-Adding a teaspoon of chia seeds to the juice will give it an extra nutrient boost.

-If you are looking for thicker juice, add a few ice cubes to the blender before blending.

-You can also add a few mint leaves to the juice for a refreshing twist.

-If you are looking for more green juice, you can add a few celery stalks to the blender before blending.

-If you want a more flavorful juice, you can add a teaspoon of freshly grated ginger before blending.

-If you want to make the juice a bit more filling, add a scoop of your favorite protein powder to the blender before blending.

-If you don't have fresh strawberries, frozen strawberries will work just as well.

-If you are looking for a creamy texture, add a few tablespoons of Greek yogurt before blending.

-If you are looking for a more filling juice, add a few tablespoons of oats to the blender before blending.

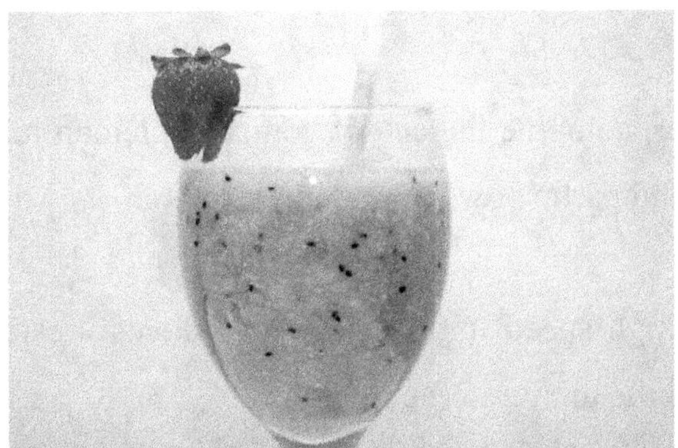

-You can replace the lime juice with orange juice for a sweeter juice.

-You can also add a few tablespoons of honey or maple syrup to the blender before blending for sweeter juice.

Celery and Tomato Juice

Ingredients:

-3 large stalks of celery, washed and roughly chopped

-2 large tomatoes, washed and roughly chopped

-1/2 cup freshly squeezed lemon juice

-1/4 teaspoon freshly ground black pepper

-1/4 teaspoon sea salt

-1/4 teaspoon garlic powder

-1 cup ice cubes

Instructions:

1. In a blender, combine the celery, tomatoes, lemon juice, pepper, salt, and garlic powder.

2. Blend on high speed until all the ingredients are fully combined and the mixture is smooth.

3. Add the ice cubes and blend for an additional 30 seconds.

4. Strain the juice through a fine-mesh sieve into a glass.

5. Enjoy your celery and tomato juice!

Tips:

-You can substitute store-bought tomato juice for fresh tomatoes if desired.

-If you want to make a larger batch, simply double or triple the ingredients.

-For a sweeter juice, add a tablespoon of honey or agave nectar.

-If you prefer your juice to be less tart, add a tablespoon of lemon juice.

-You can also add other vegetables such as carrots, bell peppers, or cucumbers for a more nutritious juice.

-If you don't have a blender, you can use a food processor or a hand blender.

-Serve your celery and tomato juice immediately for the best taste.

-This juice can also be stored in an airtight container for up to 3 days in the refrigerator.

-You can also freeze the juice for up to 3 months.

-Enjoy your celery and tomato juice with a light salad for a healthy and refreshing meal.

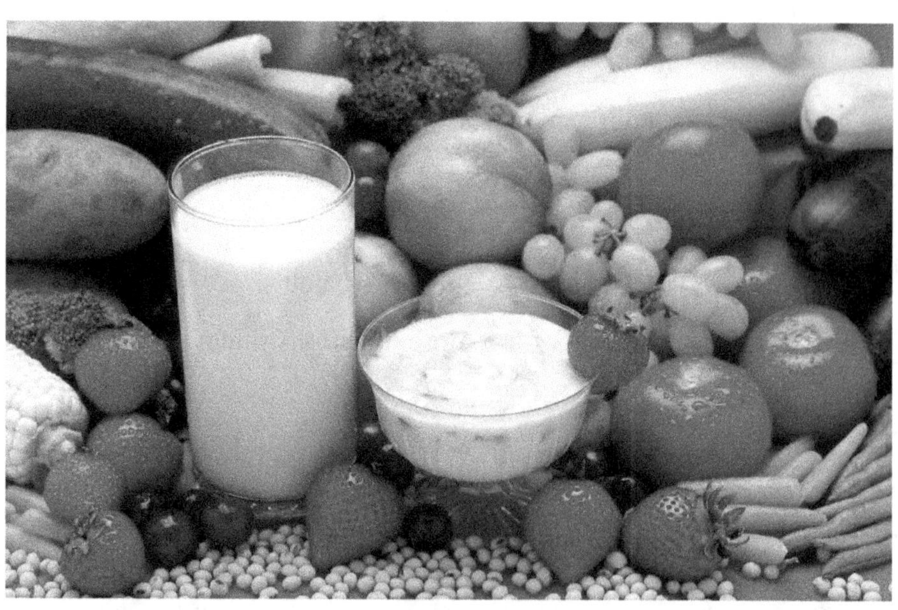

Melon and Cucumber Juice

Ingredients:

-1 medium-sized melon

-1 medium-sized cucumber

-1/2 lemon

-Ice cubes

Instructions:

1. Cut the melon in half and remove the seeds. Cut the melon into pieces, then place them into a blender.

2. Peel the cucumber and cut it into small cubes. Add the cucumber pieces to the blender.

3. Squeeze the juice from the lemon half into the blender.

4. Add a few ice cubes to the blender and blend all the ingredients until the desired consistency is reached.

5. Pour the juice into a glass and serve immediately.

Tips:

-If you like a sweeter juice, add a teaspoon of honey or agave nectar to the blender.

-For a more refreshing drink, add a few mints leaves to the blender.

-If you want an even creamier texture, add a few tablespoons of yogurt to the blender.

-For a more nutritious juice, add a handful of spinach to the blender.

-If you want a thicker consistency, add a few tablespoons of chia seeds to the blender.

-If you want to make a large batch of juice, double or triple the ingredients.

-If you want an even more refreshing drink, add a few slices of frozen fruit to the blender.

-If you want to make a smoothie, add a few tablespoons of plant-based milk to the blender.

-If you want to make a spicier drink, add a few slices of jalapeño peppers to the blender.

-If you want to make a more filling drink, add a few tablespoons of oats to the blender.

-For a healthier version, replace the ice cubes with frozen melon and cucumber cubes.

-If you want to make the juice more vibrant, add a few drops of food coloring to the blender.

-If you want to add more flavor, try adding a pinch of sea salt, ginger, or cinnamon to the blender.

Enjoy your healthy and delicious melon and cucumber juice!

Apple and Ginger Juice

Ingredients:

-4 Apples, cored and cut into wedges

-1 inch piece of fresh ginger, peeled and cut into small chunks

-1/4 cup of freshly squeezed lemon juice

-1/4 cup of water

-1/4 cup of sugar (optional)

Instructions:

1. In a blender, combine the apple wedges, ginger chunks, lemon juice, and water. Blend until the mixture is smooth.

2. If the mixture is too tart, add the sugar and blend until dissolved.

3. Strain the mixture through a sieve to remove any solids.

4. Pour the juice into glasses and serve.

Tips:

-For a sweeter juice, add more sugar.

-If you prefer a thicker juice, add some ice cubes to the blender before blending.

-For spicier juice, add a pinch of ground cayenne pepper.

-To make a larger batch, simply double or triple the ingredients.

-For a different flavor, try adding a few slices of fresh ginger to the juice.

-For a different flavor, try adding a few slices of fresh pineapple to the juice.

-To make the juice colder, add some ice cubes before serving.

-For a healthy twist, try adding a few slices of cucumber to the juice.

-For a more intense flavor, try adding a few slices of fresh mint to the juice.

-For a more tropical flavor, try adding a few slices of fresh mango to the juice.

-For a more creamy juice, try adding a few tablespoons of plain yogurt to the juice.

-For an adult twist, try adding a splash of vodka to the juice.

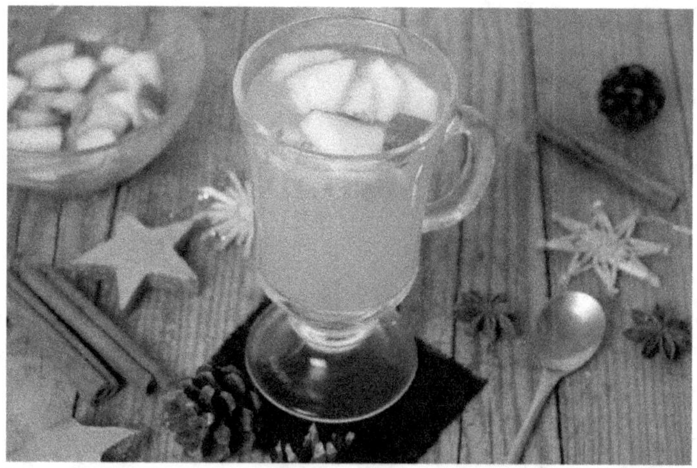

-For a healthier option, try using unsweetened almond milk instead of water and omit the sugar.

Beetroot and Green Apple Juice

Ingredients:

- 2 medium beetroots

- 2 medium green apples

- 1/2 lemon

- 1 cup of ice

Instructions:

1. Peel and dice the beetroots and place them in a blender.

2. Peel and dice the green apples and add them to the blender.

3. Squeeze the lemon juice into the blender.

4. Blend the ingredients until smooth.

5. Add a cup of ice and blend for an additional 30 seconds.

6. Strain the juice into glasses.

7. Enjoy!

Tips:

- For a sweeter juice, add a teaspoon of honey or agave syrup to the blender.

- For a more intense flavor, add a few dashes of ground ginger or cinnamon to the blender.

- If you want thicker juice, add a banana to the blender.

- For a more refreshing drink, add a few sprigs of mint to the blender.

- For a tangier flavor, add a tablespoon of lime juice to the blender.

- To make the juice colder, add a few cubes of frozen fruit to the blender.

- To make the juice creamier, add a few ice cubes and a tablespoon of yogurt to the blender.

- To make the juice more colorful, add a few slices of strawberries or blueberries to the blender.

- For an extra boost of vitamins, add a tablespoon of wheatgrass or spirulina to the blender.

- To make the juice smoother, strain it through a fine mesh strainer.

- To make the juice more filling, add a tablespoon of chia seeds to the blender.

- To make the juice more nutritious, add a tablespoon of flaxseeds or almond butter to the blender.

- For a fun twist, add a few drops of flavored extract to the blender.

- For a unique flavor, try adding a few slices of fresh ginger or turmeric root to the blender.

- To make the juice more refreshing, add a few slices of cucumber to the blender.

- To make the juice more savory, try adding a few slices of bell peppers or carrots to the blender.

- To make the juice more energizing, add a scoop of protein powder to the blender.

Kiwi and Strawberry Juice

Ingredients:

- 2 kiwis, peeled and sliced

- 8-10 strawberries, hulled and sliced

- 2 tablespoons of freshly squeezed lemon juice

Instructions:

1. Place the sliced kiwis and strawberries in a blender.

2. Add the lemon juice and blend until the mixture is smooth.

3. Strain the mixture through a sieve to remove any large chunks.

4. Pour the juice into a glass and enjoy.

Tips:

- You can add a teaspoon of honey for extra sweetness.

- If you want a thicker consistency, add some crushed ice before blending.

- For a more intense flavor, you can replace the lemon juice with lime juice.

- You can also use frozen kiwis and strawberries to make a smoothie-like drink.

- If you don't have a sieve, you can use a cheesecloth to strain out the larger chunks.

- Try adding a few mint leaves for a refreshing twist.

- Add a splash of your favorite sparkling water for a bubbly twist.

- Add a few pieces of fresh fruit to your glass for a colorful presentation.

- You can store your Kiwi and Strawberry Juice in the refrigerator for up to a week.

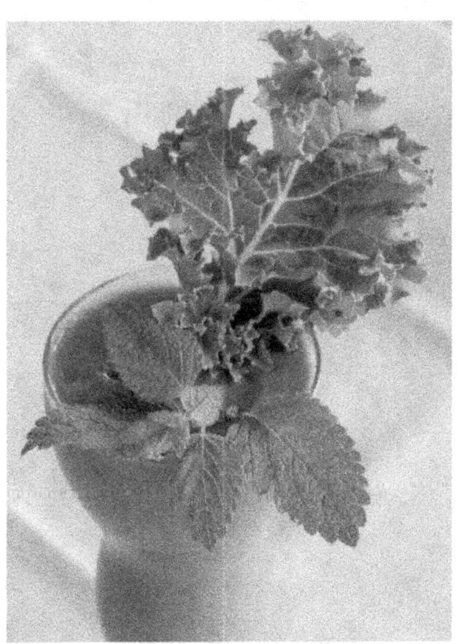

Carrot and Mango Juice

Ingredients:

- 4 carrots

- 2 mangoes

- 1 inch of fresh ginger

- 2 cups of water

Instructions:

1. Wash the carrots, mangoes, and ginger. Peel and roughly chop the carrots and mangoes.

2. Place the carrots, mangoes, and ginger into a blender.

3. Add 2 cups of water to the blender.

4. Blend the ingredients until smooth.

5. Strain the juice through a fine mesh strainer or cheesecloth.

6. Pour the juice into a glass and enjoy!

Tips:

- For an extra boost of flavor, add a pinch of turmeric, cinnamon, or cayenne pepper.

- You can also add a squeeze of lemon or lime juice to the juice.

- If you'd like a sweeter juice, add a bit of honey or agave nectar.

- To make the juice more filling, add a few ice cubes.

- If you'd like a thicker juice, add a few tablespoons of oat milk or almond milk.

- You can also freeze the juice in an ice cube tray and add the cubes to a glass of sparkling water for a refreshing and hydrating drink.

- For a frothy juice, add the juice to a blender and blend until frothy.

- If you'd like a creamier juice, add a few tablespoons of yogurt.

- Add a few fresh mint leaves for a refreshing twist.

- For a bit of crunch, add some chia or hemp seeds.

- For an extra healthy boost, add a tablespoon of spirulina or matcha powder.

- If you'd like a sweeter and more tropical juice, add a few slices of pineapple or a banana.

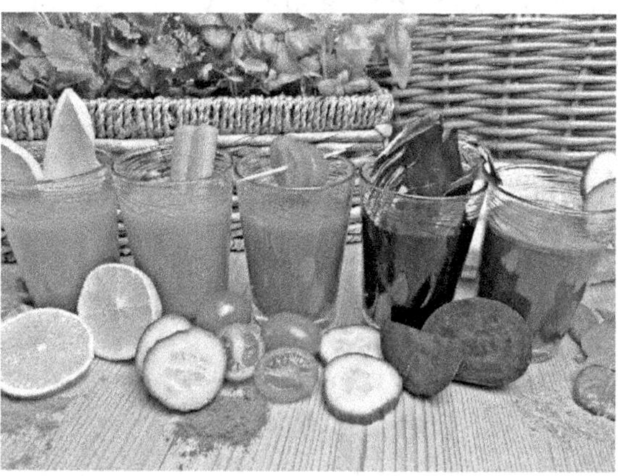

- If you'd like a more intense flavor, add a few tablespoons of freshly squeezed orange juice.

Cucumber mint juice

Ingredients:

-2 cups of cucumber, peeled and chopped

-1/2 cup of fresh mint leaves

-1/4 cup of fresh lime juice

-1/4 cup of honey (or to taste)

-2 cups of cold water

-Ice cubes (optional)

Instructions:

1. In a blender, combine cucumber, mint, lime juice, and honey.

2. Blend until smooth and all ingredients are combined.

3. Pour the mixture into a pitcher.

4. Add cold water and stir to combine.

5. Place the pitcher in the refrigerator for at least 30 minutes to allow the flavors to blend.

6. Strain the mixture into a glass over ice cubes (optional) and enjoy.

Tips:

-For a thicker juice, use less water.

-For a sweeter juice, add more honey.

-If you don't have fresh mint leaves, you can use dried mint leaves. Just add a teaspoon of dried mint leaves to the mixture and blend until smooth.

-If you don't have fresh lime juice, substitute it with lemon juice.

-Garnish the juice with a few slices of cucumber or lime for extra flavor and presentation.

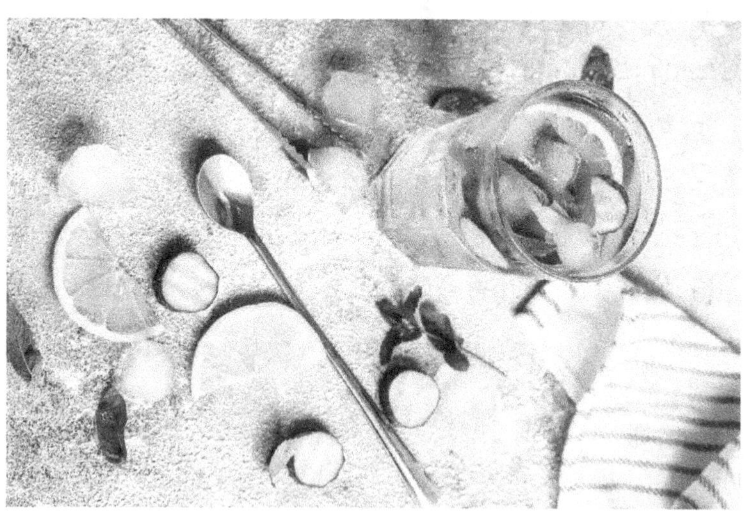

Cabbage Juice

Ingredients:

-1 head green cabbage, washed and chopped

-1 large cucumber, peeled and chopped

-1/2 apple, peeled and chopped

-2 carrots, peeled and chopped

-1/2 inch ginger root, peeled and chopped

-2 celery stalks chopped

-1/2 lemon, peeled and chopped

-1/2 teaspoon sea salt

Instructions:

1. Combine all of the chopped ingredients in a blender and blend until smooth.

2. Strain the mixture through a fine mesh sieve or cheesecloth.

3. Pour the juice into a glass and enjoy!

Tips:

-If you don't have a fine mesh sieve or cheesecloth, you can use a regular kitchen strainer to strain the mixture.

-You can also add a few ice cubes to the juice to make it cold.

-It's best to drink the juice immediately after straining, as it will start to lose its freshness over time.

-You can also add other fruits or vegetables to the juice if you like, such as beets, apples, oranges, or pineapple.

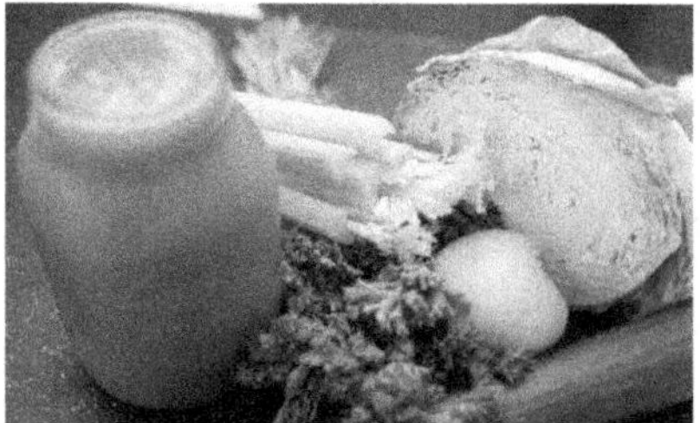

-If you don't like the taste of raw cabbage, try adding a little honey or agave syrup to the juice to sweeten it.

-Feel free to experiment with different ingredients and flavors to create your unique cabbage juice!

Skin Sustain Juice

Ingredients:

- 1 medium cucumber

- 2 large carrots

- 1/2 inch fresh ginger

- 2 oranges

- 1/2 cup fresh parsley

- 1/2 cup spinach

Instructions:

1. Wash and peel the cucumber, carrots, ginger, and oranges.

2. Slice the cucumber into thin slices and put them in the blender.

3. Peel and chop the carrots into small cubes and add them to the blender.

4. Peel and finely mince the ginger, and add it to the blender.

5. Peel the oranges and add them to the blender.

6. Add the parsley and spinach to the blender.

7. Blend all the ingredients until it forms a smooth juice.

8. Pour the juice into a glass and enjoy!

Tips:

- For a sweeter juice, you can add a teaspoon of honey or agave nectar.

- You can also add a tablespoon of flax seed oil or coconut oil for added nutritional value.

- If you're looking for a thicker consistency, you can add a few ice cubes to the blender.

- To make this juice more nutritious, you can add a handful of nuts or seeds for extra protein and healthy fats.

- You can store the juice in the refrigerator for up to 3 days.

Zucchini and Green Bean Juice

Ingredients:

-2 medium zucchinis

-2 cups green beans

-2 cups of spinach

-2 stalks of celery

-1 apple

-1 pear

-1 lemon

-1 lime

-1/2 inch of ginger

Instructions:

1. Wash and prepare all the ingredients before beginning.

2. Cut the zucchini, celery, apple, pear, lemon, and lime into small pieces.

3. Place the zucchini, green beans, spinach, celery, apple, pear, lemon, and lime into a juicer and process until smooth.

4. Peel the ginger and add it to the juicer.

5. Process until all the ingredients are blended.

6. Strain the juice through a fine mesh strainer or cheesecloth.

7. Serve chilled and enjoy!

Tips:

-If you don't have a juicer, you can use a high-speed blender and then strain the juice through a cheesecloth.

-You can adjust the number of ingredients depending on how much juice you want to make.

You can add other vegetables or fruits to the juice to make it more flavorful.

-If you want a sweeter juice, add a little bit of honey or agave syrup.

Delight Broccoli Juice

Ingredients:

-1 large bunch of broccoli

-1 large cucumber

-1 lemon

-1 teaspoon of honey

-1/2 cup of water

Instructions:

1. Wash the broccoli and cucumber thoroughly.

2. Peel the lemon and cut it into wedges.

3. Cut the broccoli into small florets and the cucumber into cubes.

4. Place the broccoli and cucumber into a high-powered blender and add the lemon wedges and honey.

5. Blend until the ingredients are completely smooth.

6. Add the water to thin out the juice and blend again.

7. Strain the juice into a glass and enjoy.

Tips:

-For a more intense flavor, you can add a few sprigs of fresh mint.

-You can also add a pinch of sea salt to balance out the sweetness of the honey.

-If you want more fiber in your juice, you can add a handful of spinach.

-If you want more sweetness, you can add an extra teaspoon of honey.

-For a creamier texture, you can add a few ice cubes.

-You can also add a few drops of fresh lime juice for a zesty flavor.

-If you want a richer flavor, you can add a scoop of fresh ginger.

-You can also add a few slices of fresh avocado for a smooth texture.

-You can use fresh or frozen broccoli for this recipe.

-If you want to make a thicker juice, you can add more broccoli.

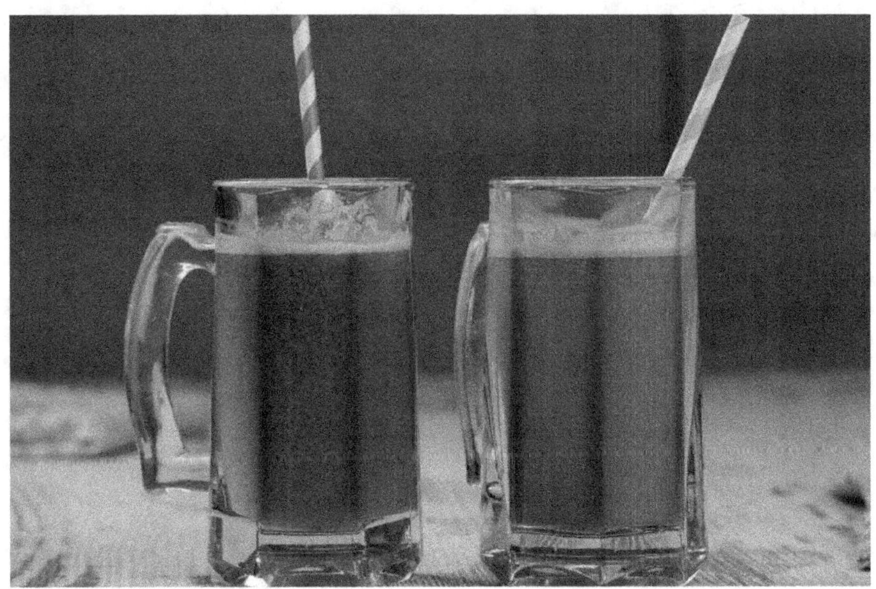

Pomegranate and Apple Juice

Ingredients:

-2 pomegranates

-2 apples

-1/4 cup freshly squeezed lemon juice

-1/4 cup honey

-4 cups cold water

Instructions:

1. Cut the pomegranates in half and scoop out the seeds. Place the pomegranate seeds into a blender.

2. Cut the apples into wedges and add them to the blender as well.

3. Add the lemon juice and honey to the blender.

4. Blend the ingredients until a smooth liquid is formed.

5. Add the cold water and blend again until everything is well combined.

6. Strain the juice through a fine-mesh sieve to remove any chunks of fruit.

7. Serve the juice chilled or over ice.

Tips:

1. To make the juice even sweeter, add an extra tablespoon of honey.

2. If you prefer a thinner consistency, add more cold water.

3. To make the juice even more nutritious, add a handful of spinach to the blender before blending.

4. If you don't have fresh pomegranates, you can also use frozen pomegranate seeds.

5. For a different flavor, try adding a pinch of ground ginger or cinnamon to the blender before blending.

6. For a more intense flavor, try adding a tablespoon of pomegranate molasses.

Green Lemonade

Ingredients:

- 2 cups freshly squeezed lemon juice

- 2 cups fresh spinach

- 2 cups fresh kale

- 2 cups fresh mint leaves

- 2 cups apple juice

- 2 cups water

- 1/2 cup honey

- 1/4 cup lime juice

Instructions:

1. Start by blending the lemon juice, spinach, kale, and mint in a blender until they are completely smooth.

2. Pour the mixture into a large pitcher or container.

3. Add the apple juice, water, honey, and lime juice to the pitcher.

4. Stir until all the ingredients are mixed.

5. Refrigerate for at least 4 hours or overnight.

6. Serve cold and enjoy!

Tips:

- You can also use frozen spinach, kale, and mint if you don't have access to fresh.

- Add a few drops of food coloring to give the lemonade a brighter green color.

- Add a few slices of lemon or lime to the pitcher for extra flavor.

- If the lemonade is too tart for your taste, add a bit more honey or lime juice.

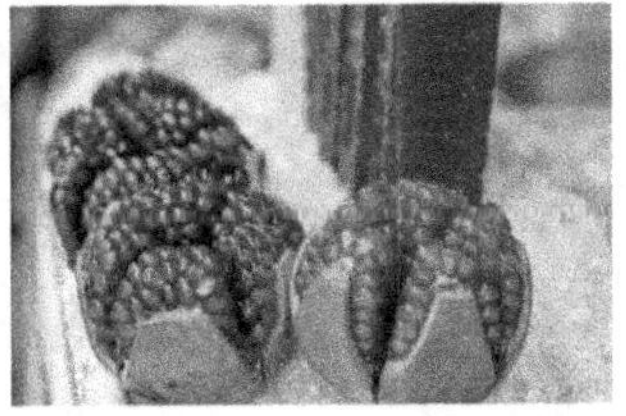

- You can also add a few slices of cucumber to the lemonade for a refreshing twist.

Beetroot and Watermelon Juice

Ingredients:

- 2 medium-sized beetroots

- 2 cups of chopped watermelon

- 1/2 cup of freshly squeezed lemon juice

- 1/2 cup of honey

- 1/2 cup of ice cubes

Instructions:

1. Start by washing the beetroots. Peel the skin and cut them into small cubes.

2. Next, add the cubes of beetroot to a blender.

3. Add the watermelon cubes and blend until the mixture reaches a smooth consistency.

4. Now, add the freshly squeezed lemon juice, honey, and ice cubes to the blender.

5. Blend again until everything is well combined.

6. Pour the juice into glasses and enjoy!

Tips:

- If you prefer a sweeter juice, you can add more honey.

- You can also add a pinch of salt to the juice for a bit of extra flavor.

- For a thinner consistency, you can add more water or a bit of coconut water.

- If you have a juicer, you can use it instead of a blender for smoother juice.

- To make this a refreshing summer drink, add some freshly chopped mint leaves.

- You can also add some pineapple juice for a tropical twist.

- For a thicker consistency, you can add some Greek yogurt or a banana.

- For a healthy twist, you can add some wheatgrass or spinach to the mix.

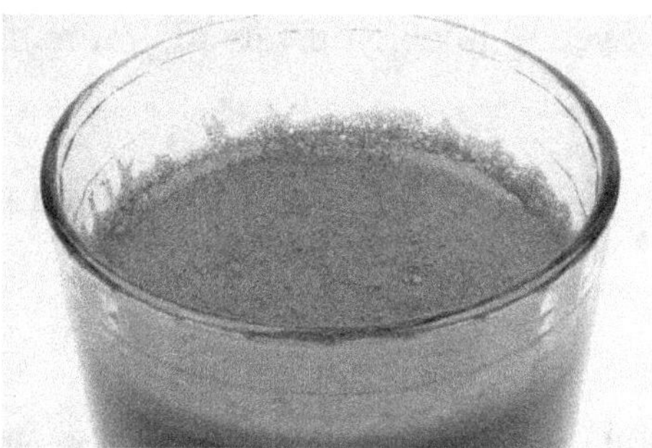

- You can also add some freshly grated ginger to the juice for a spicy kick.

- To make the juice more nutritious, add some chia or flaxseeds to the mix.

- Add some crushed ice to the juice for a cooler drink.

- For a refreshing boost, you can add a few drops of essential oils to the juice.

CONCLUSION

A thorough manual for leading a healthy and balanced life while dealing with diabetes is the ***Diabetes Juicing Cookbook***. It offers thorough instructions for making juices that are fresh and nourishing while managing diabetes and enhancing general health. Also, the book offers a wealth of knowledge on diabetes, diet, and healthy living options.

Several people with diabetes have learned how to control their disease and lead healthier lives thanks to ***The Diabetes Juicing Cookbook***. By using this book, readers can control their diabetes while savoring wonderful juices produced from fresh fruits and vegetables. For those with diabetes, the book's simple-to-follow recipes, in-depth discussion of diabetes and nutrition, and helpful suggestions for making healthy lifestyle adjustments are useful tools.

In conclusion, those who have diabetes should not be without the ***Diabetes Juicing Cookbook***. It includes delectable recipes to make it easier for people with diabetes to enjoy wholesome juices and in-depth information on diabetes and nutrition. Also feel free to leave me a mail here.

People can have scrumptious juices while controlling their diabetes and enhancing their general health by adhering to the instructions and suggestions in the book.

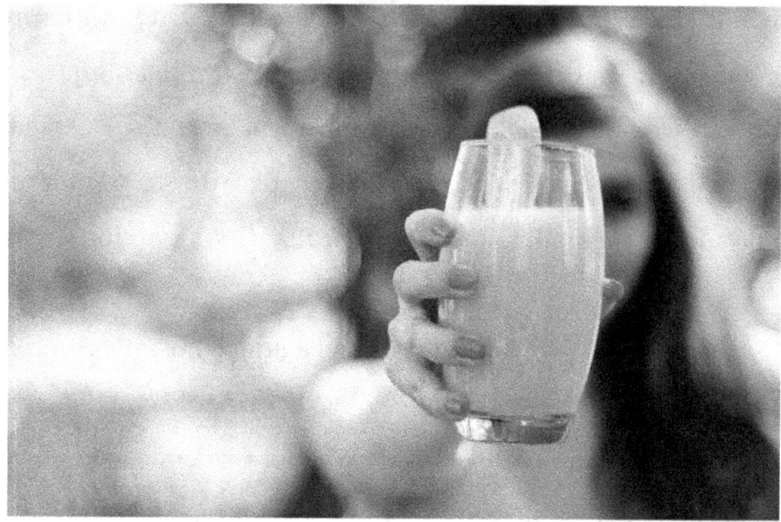

The Diabetes Juicing Cookbook is a must-have for anyone living with diabetes. It offers priceless resources and information to assist people with diabetes in learning how to control their disease and live a healthy life.